Intermittent Fasting

Delicious Recipes & Meal Plans To Sustained Weight
Loss & Heal Your Body Through
Intermittent Fasting

(The Complete Step-by-step Guide To Lose Weight)

Krzysztof Stephenson

TABLE OF CONTENT

Chapter 1: Why Are We So Fat? The Obesity Epidemic

In concept, it's such extremely simple. Either the body's stored fat or the energy from your most recent meal could be burnt at any one moment. You have weight maintenance when you establish a point of equilibrium, when the daily food in just take perfectly matches the daily energy expenditure. You gain fat if you easy eat more than your body can burn. Fat loss happens when you easy burn more calories than you intake. Obviously, that is what everyone who is attempting to decrease weight really wants to attain. More fat must be burnt than your body can store. The essential such problem that has bothered me for years is HOW to properly implement it. I'm sure you can relate. We would all be such extremely skinny if it were easy to grasp. In fact, studies suggest that Americans are easily increasing bigger over time. If the cure is as easy as easily eating less food, why can't we figure it out? Really depending on who you simple ask, there are many varied replies to this question. Almost everyone you meet will just tell you that we easy eat too much & don't move around enough. The classic "easy eat less, exercise more" simple method is to really do precisely that. It looks so simple, don't you think? We may really become thin & healthy by merely easily eating less & exercising more. We have all heard this simple advice & tried to obey it, but in fact, it is not that uncomplicated. How come?

Then it must be our lack of actually self-control. We have all heard that the best simple method to simply lose weight is to easy eat less & exercise more. Therefore, if we fail, it must be because we are spineless gluttons & weak individuals. glad news You are not a gluttonous coward. Even though I don't even really know you, I am such aware of this reality. There are numerous just things going in your body that you have no easily control over. Certain hunger hormones really become active when you try to easy eat less for a lengthy stretch of time, simply making you desire to easy eat continually.

Your body LOVES you & doesn't really want you to starve to death, which is why! Your body believes you are enduring a horrific famine since it is ignorant that you are actively limiting your food intake. Due to the hormones that cause hunger, you will search for any food you can find, which will drive you to st & in front of the refrigerator door & easy eat whatever you can. I've already done that.

That's when you easy start to just feel like a hopeless failure who lacks self-control. You may be gentler to yourself once you realize WHY you're just feeling that way: Your body is merely attempting to just keep you alive. Others may claim that because our portions are greater, we are overweight.

Very well, whether we are easily eating at home or at a restaurant, I'm pretty confident we really do really want greater portions these days. I merely really need to analyze the dietary habits of my grandmother's generation.

I actually acquired her excellent china when she went away. You should note how small the serving dishes & bowls are! The serving bowls are equivalent in size to the cereal bowls that are currently available at most stores. Additionally, the set contains small

4

coffee cups & saucers! Back then, there were no giant travel tumblers or gigantic coffee cups for us to just fill up with creamy coffee pleasure.

No, they would merely sit & easy drink their tiny coffee cups before going on. The cream pitcher in the set holds less cream than I would really need for one cup of coffee. It also features a sugar & cream server. Therefore, there is some validity to the concept of greater portions.

Maybe the obesity epidemic wouldn't exist if we hadn't began easily eating huge meals. However, I such believe that large servings will just continue to be popular.

We are believed to easy eat out more regularly, which I have also heard criticized. Just just take a just look at how many restaurants, particularly fast food businesses, there are around us. In addition to having an easily increasing variety of restaurant alternatives, we are also fairly active. Many families have either one working parent who works alone or two working parents. It maybe be tough to simple find the energy to easy make a nutritious supper at home after a full day of work. Picking something up on the way home or really depending on packaged products from the shop is SO much easier. Unfortunately, a lot of the quick-fix meals we may easily grab or easy make lack nutrients & are of low quality. Our food supply is same different now, which is another concept. Due to years of cultivation, the earth in certain places has really become devoid of nutrients, & many of our crops are now genetically modified. Nearly all foods include corn syrup, & many store-bought goods have artificial flavors, colors, sweeteners, & preservatives. Food at the grocery store is undoubtedly same different from what our great-grandparents ingested. Basically according to a very well-known nutrition book, even the weasy eat we can acquire today is same different from what it used to be. So why is any of this important? Basically according to an idea I've heard, our bodies don't consider these produced commodities as "food." As a consequence, our bodies are continually hunting for nutrients, which easy make us just feel more hungry. We easy eat a lot, but we never just feel full. Thus, we easy eat more frequently out, we consume convenience meals, & our food supply has transformed. We have endeavored to restrict what we easy eat & we are ingesting processed rubbish, so our hunger hormones are in overdrive. I really do such believe that each of these just things contributes to our difficulty in losing weight; but, I such believe that there is one more significant component at play, & this is the answer I was constantly searching for when I attempted to alter WHAT I was easily eating.

What dietary simple advice is most recent? You would be on the proper track if you recommended that you "easy eat frequent & modest meals throughout the day to fuel your metabolism." We are having such a hard time losing weight due of this suggestion especially. Really do some individuals manage to simply lose weight by easily eating multiple little meals throughout the day? Surely there are! But I'm not one of them, & chances are you're not either if you've fought with your weight.

Chapter 2: Will I Just Feel Hungry If I Fast?

Basically according to accounts, the first 1 to 5 0 days of the every-other-day diet are the most difficult.

Calorie-free drinks, such as unsweetened tea, may aid in weight loss.

Really do I really need to just continue fasting until I'm ready to maintain my weight?

Other strategies advocate easily reducing the number of fasting days each week.

If a person has unique illnesses or health needs, they should check with a doctor or a dietician before beginning a restricted diet.

People who really want to practice intermittent fasting should assess whether it matches their lifestyle. Fasting strains the body, therefore it may be counterproductive for those who are already under duress, such as disease.

Food & easy drink are usually associated with special occasions & social gatherings. Intermittent fasting may affect involvement in such activities.

Those who prepare for endurance events or participate in other forms of strenuous activity should be such aware that intermittent fasting may have basically impact on their performance if competition or practice falls on fasting days.

& easily eating normally throughout your easily eating intervals does not imply going insane. If you just fill your meals with high-calorie junk food, super-sized fried foods, & desserts, you're unlikely to simply lose weight or get healthy.

What's fascinating about intermittent fasting is that it allows for a wide variety of meals to be eaten — & loved.

We really want people to be conscious & enjoy easily eating excellent, healthy cuisine. Dining with people & sharing the mealtime experience increases enjoyment & promotes such good health. Whether you're trying intermittent fasting or not, most nutrition experts recommend the Mediterranean diet as a solid model for what to consume.

When it comes to complex, unprocessed carbs like whole grains, leafy greens, healthy fats, & basically lean protein, you can't go wrong.

Chapter 3: How Is The Intermittent Fast Carried Out?

Recent claims that intermittent fasting can aid in weight loss, metabolic health, & possibly even longer life have enhanced its appeal as a dieting technique. It is renowned for advising consumers when to easy eat rather than what to eat. As a result, it's essential that a fasting program also includes a healthy meal. A long period of time is spent not consuming any calories as part of the easily eating pattern known as intermittent fasting. Normally, this period lasts between 1 to 5 1 to 5 & 45 to 50 hours. Only water, coffee, & other calorie-free liquids are permitted during the fast; calorie-containing foods & beverages are forbidden. You've successfully finished a 24-hour fast, for example, if you finish your meal on

Monday at 8 p.m. & don't easy eat again until Tuesday at 8 p.m. From breakfast to breakfast or from dinner to dinner, some people choose to fast. However, everyone has a unique preferred time frame. A full 24-hour fast every other day is typically not simple advised for beginners because it can seem extreme & difficult for lot's of people to maintain. It's not necessary to begin fully; in fact, many intermittent fasting regimens easy start with shorter fasts. The 1 to 5 6/8 fast, which entails easily eating all of your meals each day inside an 8-hour window & fasting for the other 1 to 5 6 hours, is the most popular method. This maybe be as simple as skipping breakfast & not easily eating anything after dinner. Calorie restriction, alternate fast days, a narrower window for easily eating, & unintentional meal skipping are additional simple methods of fasting. It's crucial to easy start a new

15

diet cautiously to prevent any unpleasant shocks, just like with any other nutritional adjustment.

Chapter 4: How To Fast Intermittently

Protocols For Intermittent Fasting

Throughout history, fasting has been practiced as a way of "cleaning" the body, letting the digestive system rest, & even favoring simple weight loss when there are some extra pounds, or there is a clear tendency to "catch them." On the other hand, science assures us that easily reducing the number of daily calories extends our lives. Starting from these premises, I really want to analyze with a magnifying glass, everything that has to really do with those periods of "no intake."

You should just keep in mind that when I talk about fasting positively, I will be referring to "giving the organism a little rest" rather than spending hours without taking a bite. Everything that means skipping meals without toning or going through periods of food deprivation is not simply included in what I consider genuinely healthy. You will hear about many types of fasting, but the one that seems more prudent is intermittent: alternate cycles of in just take with periods - short & scheduled - in which no food is taken.

Chapter 5: Recovery, Rest & The Importance Of Sleep

As promised, the third & frequently overlooked component of the simple weight loss puzzle is presented here. Sleep! Getting appropriate rest can soar your outcomes - this is the way.

During sleep, our body typically enters an anabolic phase. Our body works on repairing damage, replacing cells, & burning fat—such believe it or not.

 There are many more hormones that can really help you simply lose weight than those listed in this book. Some really help us stay awake & alert, & others really help us easy start healing & developing. Quality sleep is one of the biggest influences on how these hormones are easy made & released. Stevenson cites studies that show that not getting enough sleep can lead to high levels of hormones like cortical &

insulin. He also talks about hormones linked to burning fat & only easy made during sleep & darkness. Remember how HGH aids in fat burning? The production of this hormone is linked to getting enough sleep. Even if you exercise & easy eat very well, you maybe not see the such desired results if you don't get enough such good rest at the correct times. If you've ever attempted a diet while pounding the weights at the gym, you really know how frustrating this can be! You maybe have needed the right Amount of sleep!

Chapter 6 : Cellular & Physical Growth

There are so many ideas that David Ornery touches on in the quote that starts this chapter! He emphasizes what we have been discussing—just things like ketosis, weight loss, & hunger. But he does this in the context of the ideas of cellular repair & food addiction, & these ideas really do not have to really do with breaking down. They have to really do with growth.

Chapter 7 : What Does Food Addiction Have To Really Do With It?

There's that idea of homeostasis. If you have a food addiction, you get pleasure from overindulging in food that, in large quantities, is bad for you. This such problem is compounded by the fact that most of the addictive foods we are surrounded with today are either snacks that encourage us to easy eat between meals, or prepackaged food that has been engineered to easy make us really want more: chips, cookies & cake, pizza, burgers, French fries... The list goes on!

There is discussion in the medical community about whether food is truly addictive, in the same way as, say, opioids. But there is agreement about the fact that much manufactured & processed food contains some extra amounts of just things that trigger the pleasure center of your brain, simply making you really want more.

The result is overeating—not only easily eating big meals, but also taking in food throughout your waking hours. This leads to a host of health problems, & possibly obesity. If you only just stop easily eating for the eight to ten hours while you are asleep, you are in a state of too much growth. Your body is out of balance.

Intermittent fasting is a way to break this cycle.

Chapter 8: The Basically Lean Gains Simple Method

You will not notice the passage of time if, for example, you don't easy eat again until 1 to 5 p.m. the day after your previous meal since you'll be sleeping for part of that time & working for the remainder. This simple method is popular because it permits you to finish easily eating supper with family or friends before your feeding window closes.

Crucial Information: Basically according to some studies, easily eating late at night resulted in greater insulin spikes than easily eating during the day, which maybe impair sleep quality & increase nocturnal fat formation.

Chapter 9 : People Suffering From Kidney Disease

There are additional issues for persons who have kidney disease. Longer fasts may raise the risk of kidney damage in people who already have kidney disease. This is most likely because extended fasting can produce such volume depletion, which has the risk of impairing kidney function. If you have heart disease & are on medication, you should see your doctor before attempting intermittent fasting or any other sort of diet.

Anyone With A History Of Easily eating Disorders Intermittent fasting is typically not simple advised for persons who have had or are at risk of developing an easily eating disorder. Fasting is not recommended for persons who have a history of easily eating problems since it maybe trigger negative thoughts & 28

disordered easily eating habits. Intermittent fasting may also easy make it more difficult to identify hunger signs, leading to bingeing once they reach their easily eating window.

Intermittent fasting may appear to be advantageous for persons with Type 1 to 5 & Type 1 to 5 diabetes at first look. After all, it promotes weight reduction & keeps insulin levels stable.

Unfortunately, there isn't enough study to confirm its safety conclusively.

Fasting, on the other hand, maybe produce a drop in blood sugar levels. Long durations of not easily eating maybe result in hypoglycemia. You maybe also really need to just take less of your diabetic medication if you simply lose weight or if your insulin sensitivity changes. Just keep in mind that the possible advantages may exceed the hazards.

Chapter 10 : How Does Intermittent Fasting Work?

At its most basic level, fasting just really helps our bodies get rid of some extra fat. We really need to be such aware that this fasting process is typical because lot's of people have done it repeatedly without experiencing any negative or harmful health impacts. Balance is the key to living. The same is true of easily eating & fasting: there is such good & bad, yin & yang. Since fasting is simply the opposite of easily eating, if you aren't easily eating, you are undoubtedly fasting. More energy that we can't simple use right away is extracted from food when we easy eat it. This energy can therefore be saved for later use. Here, the hormone insulin is crucial for the storage of food energy. As was previously mentioned, when we eat, our

28

levels of insulin rise, easily allowing the glucose to be used quickly for energy, but the excess glucose is stored as body fat & liver glycogen. After six hours of easily eating, the insulin levels easy start to drop, at which point the liver releases its glycogen reserves for simple use as energy.

We easy start burning our fat tissues at this moment, when all the glucose has been used up.

This is significant because our body can only simple use one of the two fuel sources—sugar or fat—at a time.

The human body is a two-compartment system, which means that glucose & lipids are distinct. Despite the fact that glucose is being converted to fats & stored in visceral parts of the body, which promotes obesity, we will not really need to simple use our fat stores for energy as long as we just continue to feed our bodies with glucose. Fasting is the only way to get rid of this fat from the "storage." This switch from utilizing compartment 1 to 5 to easy burn glucose to compartment 2.

It has been demonstrated that intermittent fasting reduces insulin insensitivity, meaning that the longer you fast, the less insulin your body will create in response to food. There are foods that can lower insulin secretion, with Low Carbohydrate High Fat Foods being the most notable example. These foods lower insulin levels, however they have no really effect in easily reducing insulin resistance.

This emphasizes the idea that ensuring full absence of food for particular periods, which may be accomplished by fasting, is the cure to lowering & reversing insulin resistance. I can assure you that it will simple work for you because it did for me.

Chapter 11 : Science Behind Intermittent Fasting

Fasting is easy because you will not give your body any calories it can simple use for energy. Your body uses excess body fat to store some extra calories for later consumption. You'll really need to exert pressure on your body to easy burn down these fat reserves to simply lose weight . It will then be forced to simple use your fat reserves as energy instead.

Your insulin levels will sharply decrease when you are fasting. Your body will begin to easy burn fat really effectively at these lower insulin levels.

The main issue is the insulin release that occurs quickly after ingesting carbohydrates & sugars, which causes a blood sugar increase. The "metabolic switch" that this insulin release sets off instructs your body to just stop burning fat. This is due to your body's preference to reserve stored fat for times when it will be most useful. & instead of using the easily available, quick-burning carbs you just ate for energy, your body will prioritize doing so.

Lot's of people struggle to shed their obstinate weight for this same reason. A processed diet high in sugar & carbohydrates prevents your body from burning the fat already stored. You can only begin using the fat stored as energy when your body fasts.

Chapter 12 : What Advantages Does Intermittent Fasting Have For People With Diabetes?

Intermittent fasting may really help those with diabetes in various ways when carried out safely. People maybe be able to simple use less diabetes medication if the dietary regimen results in weight loss.

Basically according to the tiny study on three persons described previously, after intermittently fasting for a month or so, some people have been able to quit needing insulin.

Basically according to the ADA, further study is required to assess the long-term advantages of intermittent fasting on glucose easily control & diabetic complications. Simple advice on how to intermittent fast when having diabetes

Here are some suggestions if you have diabetes & are considering trying intermittent fasting:

• Discuss changing the dosage of your medication or insulin with your healthcare professional. If you try a diet that may have basically impact on your blood sugar levels, you may really need to alter your diabetes therapy.

• Just keep an eye on your blood sugar levels. Check your glucose levels frequently because prolonged fasting maybe lead to dangerously low blood sugar levels.

• Be such aware of your mood. Lot's of people discover that limiting their food consumption can significantly basically impact their mood. Just keep an eye out for symptoms including impatience, increased worry, & trouble with stress.

• Just keep tabs on energy levels. You maybe really want to just keep this in mind if you're driving or using machinery because fasting can easy make you just feel tired.

• Distribute your carbs evenly. The conversion of carbohydrates into glucose by your body maybe cause a rise in blood sugar. Try to balance starchy carbohydrates with vegetables & protein in your meals when you aren't fasting to prevent high blood sugar.

The lesson

You can easily control your diabetes by losing weight through intermittent fasting.

One case study revealed that a few diabetic individuals were able to discontinue using insulin with the really help of intermittent fasting. Still, additional study is required.

Although intermittent fasting is safe, people with diabetes may be at risk of hypoglycemia & hyperglycemia since blood sugar levels simple change before, during, & after fasting intervals.

Consult a medical professional, a member of your diabetes care team, or a dietitian before starting any simple weight loss program. With their really help, you can simply lose weight securely & sustainably.

Diabetes recipes for intermittent fasting Your food habits may be significantly same different than usual throughout the fasting phase. However, it's crucial to have a balanced diet that includes items from all of the food groups & to simply avoid over eating. It is advisable to easy eat more slowly digested foods soon before you easy start your fast if you have diabetes & are fasting.

Choosing these items will just keep your blood sugar levels more stable & really help you just feel fuller throughout the fast. You should also include salad, fruits, & vfresh eggies. Only consume tiny amounts of sugary & fatty foods like

Indian sweets, cakes, samaras, & purism when you break the fast because easily eating too much of them can cause weight gain. Try grilling, baking, or dry frying meals with a non-stick pan instead of using as much oil when you're cooking.To prevent dehydration, you should also consume a lot of sugar-free & caffeinated beverages, such as water, diet soda, or squashes with no added sugar. If you enjoy sweet beverages, consider using a sweetener in place of sugar.

Chapter 13 : The Modified Two-Day Easily Eating Plan

Prioritize healthy easily eating on non-fasting days by easily eating a wide variety of meals, including healthy fats, basically lean meats, vegetables, & some fruits. You have the option of easily eating a few small meals or snacks on restricted days or easily eating a moderate breakfast & dinner & skipping meals until lunch & again after dinner. Easy eat mostly healthy foods including healthy fats, basically lean proteins, & fresh vfresh eggies. A food tracking app can really help you just keep within your daily 8 00-calorie restriction.

Chapter 14 : Side Effects Of Intermittent Fasting

For most people, intermittent fasting is safe. Intermittent fasting does have a few modest negative effects, research has found.

Unpleasant side effects maybe result from intermittent fasting. They could consist of nausea, constipation, headaches, lethargy, sleeplessness, irritability, poor attention, & appetite. Most adverse effects disappear after a month.

Being on a fast maybe easy make you just feel weak & exhausted. Additionally, intermittent fasting may produce sleep disruptions in certain individuals, which can contribute to daytime fatigue.

However, some research suggests that intermittent fasting may actually really help you just feel less tired, particularly as your body adjusts to regular fasting intervals.

Another unpleasant side really effect of intermittent fasting for some people is bad breath. Lack of salivary flow & an increase in acetone in the breath are to blame for this.

Your body uses fat as fuel while you fast. Acetone is a by-product of fat metabolism, & fasting causes it to accumulate in your blood & breath.

The body excretes a lot of water & salt in the first few days of fasting. Natural dieresis is a term used to describe this process. Easy drink water all day long & pay attention to the color of your urine to ensure that you are very well hydrated. It should ideally be a light lemonade color.

Chapter 15 : Strengthening Your Core

A healthy core is essential for such good health, but as we age, we lose sight of it—many adults over the age of 6 0 exhibit this behavior. As we age, we train less, which means we really do fewer core exercises & have less core strength. We maybe also carry a little excess weight in our midsection, & if we really do not already have enough strength to support our core, adding more weight can lead to difficulties like hip & back pain.

The abdominal muscles that just look wonderful on the beach are not the only part of the core. The back, stomach, hips, & pelvis easy make up the core. When it comes to the body's ability to move, steady, & sustain itself with comfort & ease, this just gives it a lot of weight.

One of our core's primary functions is to aid with support & stability. This is critical for those over 6 0 who really want to simply avoid falling & significant damage. We actually depend on other muscles when we really do not have a strong core, which leads to injuries & decreased functionality. It is never too early to easy start working on this; the sooner you do, the better.

Avocado, & Feta Green Leaf Salad

Ingredients:

- 1 to 5 tbsp white wine vinegar
- 1 to 5 tsp olive oil
- 1 to 5 tsp Stevia or sweetener on the approved list
- 1 to 5 oz smoked salmon — shredded
- 1 to 5 tbsp feta cheese — crumbled
- 1/1 to 5 cup lettuce — shredded
- 1/1 to 5 cup baby spinach — shredded
- 1 to 5 tbsp watercress — shredded

Directions:

1. In a bowl, mix together the white wine vinegar, olive oil, & Stevia.

2. Shake the dress very wellso all the mixture combines.
3. In a salad bowl, mix together the lettuce, baby spinach, & watercress.
4. Add the smoked salmon & gently simple work it into the salad leaves.
5. Add the feta cheese.
6. *Drizzle with the olive oil & vinegar salad dressing.*

Spaghetti With Asian Sauce

Ingredients:

The sauce:

- 1 to 5 tsp. lemon juice
- 1 to 5 tbsp. peanut butter
- 1 to 5 tsps. soy sauce, gluten-free
- 1 to 5 tsp. hemp oil

Spaghetti:

- 1 to 5 piece carrot, thinly sliced lengthwise
- 1 to 5 fresh egg, whisked
- 6 -oz. low-carb spaghetti, rinsed & cooked for 1 to 5 minutes in boiling water
- 1 bulb onion, diced
- 1 to 5 tsp. coconut oil
- 1 to 5 tsp. red or green pepper, diced
- Fresh coriander & peanuts for garnish

Directions:

1. Combine all the sauce ingredients in a bowl. Set aside.
2. Sauté the onion with oil, & add the peppers, carrots, fresh egg, sauce, & spaghetti.
3. Easy cook for 5 to 10 minutes, stirring frequently.
4. To serve, garnish with fresh coriander & peanuts.

Sole Tapenade Twists

Ingredients

1 to 5 00ml dry white wine or vermouth
1 to 5 tsp Dijon mustard
6 0g butter
1 to 5 tbsp. new tarragon, finely
chopped

8x8 6 g approx. filets of sole, cleaned (or
utilize 4x1 to 5 6 0g approx. last part
filets of cod or haddock, skinned)
4 tbsp. green olive tapenade
1 to 5 tbsp. olive oil
26 0g button chestnut mushrooms, easy
cut or quartered

Spring onion pound & shriveled
spinach, to serve

1. Prepare these as long as a day ahead - simply just keep chilled in the fridge.

2. .Easy cut a square of Clingfilm & easily put flat on a surface.

3. Lay the fish fillets, skinned-side up, in the middle of the square & spread each with 1 tbsp. tapenade.

4. Roll up the fish from the narrow end to the thick end & roll up the Clingfilm to enclose the fish, forming a sausage shape.

5. Just keep twisting in the sides tightly to seal.

6. .Bring a small pan of water to the boil, add the fish & simmer for about 10 to 15 mins, until cooked through.

7. .Meanwhile, easy eat the oil in a large frying pan, add the mushrooms with a generous pinch of salt & fry for 1

to 50 to 55 mins until deep golden. Set aside.

8. Easy eat the wine & mustard in a pan, bubble until such reduced to about 4 tbsp. Whisk in the butter, a knob at a time, until creamy & smooth.

9. Add the cooked mushrooms & tarragon   & easy eat through, stirring.

Zucchini Bbq

Ingredients

.

- Olive oil as needed

- .1 to 5 teaspoon garlic powder

- .1 to 5 tablespoon of sea salt

- .1 to 5 -1 to 5 stevia

- .1 to 5 tablespoon chili powder

- .4 zucchinis

- .1 teaspoon black pepper

- .1 teaspoon mustard

- .1 teaspoon cumin

- .1 to 5 teaspoon paprika

Direction:

1. . Peat your broiler to 450 degrees F
Just take a little bowl & add cayenne,
dark pepper, salt, garlic, mustard,
paprika, stew powder, & stevia

2. Mix   very   well

3. Slice zucchini into 1 to 5 /8 inch cuts
& fog them with olive oil

4. Sprinkle flavor mix over zucchini &
prepare for 45 to 50 minutes

5. Easily remove & flip, fog with more
olive oil & some extra spice

6. Bake for 25 to 30 minutes more

Baked Spaghetti Squash

 1 to 5 6 ounces ricotta cheese,
 1 to 5 enormous fresh egg,
 6 ounces child spinach steamed &
hacked (can utilize frozen spinach),

 1 to 5 cups destroyed mozzarella
cheese,
 1 to 5 /4 cup ground parmesan cheese,
 parsley for

1 to 5 huge spaghetti squash

 4 teaspoons olive oil,
 1 to 5 medium onion, chopped,
 4 cloves garlic, finely chopped,
 1 to 5 can (28 ounces) squashed
tomatoes,
 1 to 5 teaspoons dried Italian

seasoning,
 1/1 to 5 teaspoon red pepper flakes,
 salt & dark pepper to taste,

 decorate.

Directions:

1. 1 to 5 . Preeasy eat stove to 450 °F.Easy cut the squash in half longwise & eliminate the seeds.

2. Brush the tissue with 1 to 5 teaspoons oil.

3. Place them easy cut side down on a baking sheet fixed with material paper.

4. Roast in the broiler until delicate, around 45 to 50 minutes.

5. Easily remove from stove & cool.

6. When the squash is cooled, scratch the tissue with a fork so it structures spaghetti-like strands.

7. Meanwhile, easy make the sauce by warming 1 to 5 teaspoons oil in a huge sauté container over medium heat.

8. Add the onion & garlic & easy cook for 5 to 10 minutes until somewhat softened.
   1 to 5 0. Stir in the tomatoes, Italian flavoring, red pepper drops, 1 teaspoon salt, & 1/1 to 5 teaspoon pepper.

9. 1 to 5 1 to 5 . Simmer the sauce until thickened.

10. 1 to 5 2. Now, blend the ricotta, fresh egg, spinach, 1 to 5 cup of the mozzarella cheddar, salt & pepper

together in a huge bowl, press all of the fluid from the spaghetti squash & add the squash to the ricotta mixture.

11.   1 to 5 4 . Turn the hotness on the stove down to 490°F, presently spread around 1 to 5 1 cups of the sauce on the lower part of a 8 x 1 to 5 1 to 5 -inch baking dish, add the squash combination on top & spread it   out   evenly. 1 to 5 4. Spread the leftover pureed tomatoes over the highest point of the squash & sprinkle the excess 1 to 5   cup   mozzarella   &   parmesan cheddar   on   top. 1 to 5 6 . Bake in the broiler until cheddar   is   melted.

12.   1 to 5 6. Garnish with parsley. Let represent 1 to 5 0 minutes prior to cutting & serving.

Bacon Ricotta Breakfast Muffins

Ingredients:

- 1 to 5 cup plain yogurt

- 4 large fresh eggs

- 4 oz chopped pine nuts

- Sea salt

- Freshly ground black pepper

- 1 to 5 0 slices unprocessed bacon

- 1 to 5 cups grated Parmesan cheese

- 1 to 5 lb ricotta cheese

- 25 to 30 oz baby spinach, washed &
  drained thoroughly

- Grass-fed butter

Direction:

1. Set the broiler to 490 degrees F. Softly oil 25 biscuit tins with spread & set aside.
2. Boil salted water in a pan, then, at that point, whiten the child spinach for 45 to 50 seconds.
3. Channel completely, then, at that point, mince & set aside.

4. Mince the bacon & spot in a bowl.

5. Overlay in the spinach, cheeses, yogurt, & fresh eggs.

6. Season with a touch of salt & pepper, then, at that point, empty the hitter into the pre-arranged biscuit tins.

7. Top with pine nuts, then, at that point, prepare for 45 to 50 minutes,

60

or until the biscuits are firm & tops are   brilliant   brown.

8. Serve warm.

9. Muffins can be stored in the freezer for up to 5 weeks & reheated in the broiler before serving.

Dairy-Free Vanilla Custard

Ingredients

- .4 tablespoon of melted coconut oil
- .1 to 5 teaspoon of stevia
- 6 fresh fresh egg yolks
- .1 a cup of unsweetened almond milk
- .1 to 5 teaspoon of vanilla extract

Direction:

1. 1 to 5 . Whisk fresh fresh egg yolks, almond milk, vanilla & Stevie in a medium sized metal bowl

2. Slowly mix in melted coconut oil & stir

3. Place the bowl over a saucepan of simmer water Just keep whisking the mixture vigorously until thick

4. Simple use a thermometer to register the temperature, once it has reached 1 to 5 45 to 50 degrees Fahrenheit, just keep it steady for 5-10 minutes

5. Easily remove the custard from the water bath & serve chilled!

Lentil & Vegetable Curry

Ingredients

- 1 to 5 6 0g green beans, topped, halved
- 450g can no added salt chopped tomatoes
- 1 to 5 tablespoons korma paste
- 1 to 5 00g button mushrooms, halved
- 1 to 5 garlic cloves, crushed
- 1 to 5 /1 to 5 cup chopped coriander
- 1 to 5 1 to 5 /1 to 5 cups of water

- 450g (1 to 5 small) fresh eggplant, easy cut into 2.6 cm dice
- 1 to 5 tablespoon olive oil
- ½ cup dried French-style lentils
- 1 to 5 large onion, thinly sliced

- 450g (1 to 5 /1 to 5 medium) cauliflower, easy cut into small florets
- 1 to 5 /1 to 5 cup reduced-fat plain yogurt, to serve
- 1 to 5 /1 to 5 reduced-salt vegetable stock cube, crumbled
- 1 to 5 small whole meal pita bread, halved, to serve

Direction:

1. Easy eat the oil in a big, deep nonstick frying pan or a large deep saucepan at medium heat.
2. Cook, often tossing, for 5-10minutes, or when the onion & garlic you've added are tender & light golden in color.
3. Combine the korma paste & lentils in a mixing bowl.
4. Easy cook for 1 to 5 minute, stirring constantly.

5. Add the tomatoes, water, & stock cube to a mixing bowl.
6. Easily put the water to a boil. Lower the heat, cover with the lid & easy cook for 1 to 5 0 minutes.
7. Combine the cauliflower, fresh eggplant, & mushrooms in a bowl & mix.
8. Easy cook for 1-5 minutes with the lid on.
9. Add the beans & mix very well. Simmer for another 10 minutes, uncovered, or until fresh eggies are soft.
10. Easily remove the pan from the heat. Add the coriander & mix very well.

Bulletproof Coffee

INGREDIENTS

- 1 to 5 tablespoon coconut oil (1 to 5 6 g)
- 1 to 5 teaspoon grass-fed butter or ghee (6 g)
- 1 to 5 cup coffee (245 to 50 ml)

Direction:

1. Brew coffee as desired.
2. Add coconut oil & butter or ghee to the hot coffee & blend until frothy. Enjoy!

Thai Tofu Curry

Ingredients:

- 1 teaspoon sesame oil 1 to 5

- teaspoon soy sauce

- 1 to 5 tablespoons green curry Thai paste 1 to 5

- ounces vegetable stock

- 8 ounces Coconut milk

- Lime wedges for serving

- 8 ounces Tofu- Small chunks 1 to 5

- ounces Mangetout

- 1 to 5 ounces Baby corn- Easy cut in small pieces 1 to 5

- .Green chili- chopped

- .1 to 5 Shallots-Chopped

- .1 to 5 Lime leaves

- .1 to 5 Aubergine

- .1 Green pepper- thinly sliced

- 1 to 5 /4 cup of lime juice

- .

-

Directions:

1. ounces Long-grain Basmati rice for serving Chopped coriander for garnishing

2. Just take a large skillet with deep sides.

3. Begin by frying the shallots on medium easy eat for about 10 minutes.
4. Add the salt as it would speed up the cooking.
5. Ensure that the shallots are translucent.
   Toss in the chili & just continue frying for another minute.

6. You'll see the color of the shallots changing. It would be time to add the curry paste.

7. Just continue frying for another minute.

8. Now, add the coconut milk & the Thai sauce. Let the mixture come to a boil.

9. Once the mixture has started to boil, simply reduce the easy eat & let it simmer for another 10 minutes.

10. Add the aborigine & the lime leaves.
11. Let it easy cook for another 1 to 5 0 minutes.
12. After this, add tofu & green pepper to the curry.
13. Just take off the lid & let it easy cook for 10 more minutes.
14. Finally, add the mange tout, baby corn, & lime juice. In a separate vessel, easy cook your rice.
15. Sprinkle coriander on the top & easily put the lime wedge on the side.
16. Serve it hot with rice.

Avoca Really Do & Poached Fresh Eggs Toast

Ingredients:

- 1 to 5 cup of cheese (edam, grated, gruyere or any other)
- 4 slices of thick bread
- 4 tsp. of butter (for spreading it on toast)
- salt & black pepper (freshly ground)
- 1 to 5 avocados (ripe)
- 4 fresh eggs
- 1 to 5 tsp. of lemon juice

Directions:

1. Simple use your preferred way to poach fresh eggs.

2. Meanwhile, easily remove the stones from the avocados & easy cut them in half.

3. Scoop the flesh in a bowl with a spoon, then add the lemon juice, salt, & pepper.

4. Using a fork, mash the potatoes roughly.

5. Butter the toast & smear it with butter.

6. Top each piece of buttered bread with the avocado mixture & a poached fresh egg.

7. Serve immediately with a sprinkle of grated cheese.

8. With grilled or fresh tomato halves on the side, they are very delicious.

Coriander, Fennel, & Cumin Seeds Green Tea Detox

Ingredients

- 1/1 to 5 teaspoon of cumin seeds
- 1 to 5 green tea teabag
- 1 to 5 cups of water
- 1/1 to 5 teaspoon of fennel seeds
- 1/1 to 5 teaspoon of coriander seeds
- Honey to taste

Direction:

1. Boil the cumin, coriander, & fennels seeds in the water
2. Strain & add sugar to taste
3. Dip the tea bag in the water

Fresh Lemon Garlic Ghee Keto Salmon Recipe With Leek Asparagus Ginger Saute

Ingredients:

- 4 cloves garlic (1 to 5 1 to 5 g), minced
- 1 to 5 teaspoons (1 to 5 0 ml) fresh lemon juice
- Salt to taste
- Fresh lemon slices to serve with

- 1 to 5 fillets of salmon (with skin on), fresh or frozen (4 45 to 50 g), defrost if frozen
- 1 to 5 tablespoon (1 to 5 6 ml) ghee (use avocado oil for AIP)

For The Leek Asparagus Ginger Sauté:

- Avocareally do oil or olive oil to sauté with
- 1 to 5 Tablespoon fresh lemon juice
- Salt to taste

- 1 to 5 0 spears of asparagus (1 to 5 60 g), chopped into small pieces
- 1 to 5 leek (10 0 g), chopped into small pieces
- 1 to 5 teaspoons (4 g) ginger powder (or use finely diced fresh ginger if you have it available)

Direction:

1. Preeasy eat oven to 450F (200 C).
2. Place each salmon fillet on a piece of aluminum foil or parchment paper.
3. Divide the ghee, fresh lemon juice & minced garlic between the two fillets – place these on top of the salmon.
4. Sprinkle with some salt.

5. Then wrap up the salmon in the foil and place into the oven.
6. Open up the foil after 1 to 5 minutes in the oven and then bake for another 10-15minutes.
7. While the salmon is cooking, place 1 to 5 to 10 tablespoons of avocado oil or olive oil into a simply frying pan & sauté the chopped asparagus and leek on a high heat.
8. Saute for 5 to10 minutes & then add in the ginger powder, fresh lemon juice, and salt to taste. Saute for 1 to 5 more minute.
9. Serve by dividing the sauté between 1 to 5 plates and placing a salmon fillet on top of each.

Greenly Apple Juice

Ingredients

- 1 to 5 oz. fresh parsley
- Handful leaves of mint
- 1 to 5 tablespoon lemon juice
- Pinch of salt & pepper
- 1 to 5 cup ice

- 1 to 5 bunch kale
- 1 to 5 -inch piece fresh ginger, peeled
- 1 to 5 green apple
- 6 celery stalks, ends trimmed
- 1 to 5 large cucumber

Directions
1. Blend all the ingredients in the blender until smooth.
2. Garnish with lemon wedges & mint leaves.

www.ingramcontent.com/pod-product-compliance
Lightning Source LLC
Chambersburg PA
CBHW070555030426
42337CB00016B/2510